I0528321

This planner belongs to:

_____

2025

January

S	M	T	W	T	F	S
			1	2	3	4
5	6	7	8	9	10	11
12	13	14	15	16	17	18
19	20	21	22	23	24	25
26	27	28	29	30	31	

February

S	M	T	W	T	F	S
						1
2	3	4	5	6	7	8
9	10	11	12	13	14	15
16	17	18	19	20	21	22
23	24	25	26	27	28	

March

S	M	T	W	T	F	S
						1
2	3	4	5	6	7	8
9	10	11	12	13	14	15
16	17	18	19	20	21	22
23	24	25	26	27	28	29
30	31					

April

S	M	T	W	T	F	S
		1	2	3	4	5
6	7	8	9	10	11	12
13	14	15	16	17	18	19
20	21	22	23	24	25	26
27	28	29	30			

May

S	M	T	W	T	F	S
				1	2	3
4	5	6	7	8	9	10
11	12	13	14	15	16	17
18	19	20	21	22	23	24
25	26	27	28	29	30	31

June

S	M	T	W	T	F	S
1	2	3	4	5	6	7
8	9	10	11	12	13	14
15	16	17	18	19	20	21
22	23	24	25	26	27	28
29	30					

July

S	M	T	W	T	F	S
		1	2	3	4	5
6	7	8	9	10	11	12
13	14	15	16	17	18	19
20	21	22	23	24	25	26
27	28	29	30	31		

August

S	M	T	W	T	F	S
					1	2
3	4	5	6	7	8	9
10	11	12	13	14	15	16
17	18	19	20	21	22	23
24	25	26	27	28	29	30
31						

September

S	M	T	W	T	F	S
	1	2	3	4	5	6
7	8	9	10	11	12	13
14	15	16	17	18	19	20
21	22	23	24	25	26	27
28	29	30				

October

S	M	T	W	T	F	S
			1	2	3	4
5	6	7	8	9	10	11
12	13	14	15	16	17	18
19	20	21	22	23	24	25
26	27	28	29	30	31	

November

S	M	T	W	T	F	S
						1
2	3	4	5	6	7	8
9	10	11	12	13	14	15
16	17	18	19	20	21	22
23	24	25	26	27	28	29
30						

December

S	M	T	W	T	F	S
	1	2	3	4	5	6
7	8	9	10	11	12	13
14	15	16	17	18	19	20
21	22	23	24	25	26	27
28	29	30	31			

Year in Pixels

	J	F	M	A	M	J	J	A	S	O	N	D
1.												
2.												
3.												
4.												
5.												
6.												
7.												
8.												
9.												
10.												
11.												
12.												
13.												
14.												
15.												
16.												
17.												
18.												
19.												
20.												
21.												
22.												
23.												
24.												
25.												
26.												
27.												
28.												
29.												
30.												
31.												

Color Codes

Notes

January

2025

MONDAY	TUESDAY	WEDNESDAY	THURSDAY
		1	2
6	7	8	9
13	14	15	16
20	21	22	23
27	28	29	30

January

2025

FRIDAY	SATURDAY	SUNDAY	NOTES
3	4	5	○
			○
			○
			○
			○
10	11	12	○
			○
			○
			○
			○
17	18	19	○
			○
			○
			○
24	25	26	○
			○
			○
			○
			○
31			NOTES

February

MONDAY	TUESDAY	WEDNESDAY	THURSDAY
3	4	5	6
10	11	12	13
17	18	19	20
24	25	26	27

February 2025

FRIDAY	SATURDAY	SUNDAY	NOTES
	1	2	○
			○
			○
			○
			○
7	8	9	○
			○
			○
			○
			○
14	15	16	○
			○
			○
			○
21	22	23	○
			○
			○
			○
			○
28			NOTES

March

2025

MONDAY	TUESDAY	WEDNESDAY	THURSDAY
		1	2
6	7	8	9
13	14	15	16
20	21	22	23
27	28	29	30

March

FRIDAY	SATURDAY	SUNDAY	NOTES
3	4	5	○
			○
			○
			○
			○
10	11	12	○
			○
			○
			○
17	18	19	○
			○
			○
			○
			○
24	25	26	○
			○
			○
			○
			○
31			NOTES

April 2025

MONDAY	TUESDAY	WEDNESDAY	THURSDAY
	1	2	3
7	8	9	10
14	15	16	17
21	22	23	24
28	29	30	

April

FRIDAY	SATURDAY	SUNDAY	NOTES
4	5	6	○
			○
			○
			○
			○
11	12	13	○
			○
			○
			○
18	19	20	○
			○
			○
			○
			○
25	26	27	○
			○
			○
			○
			○
			NOTES

May

MONDAY	TUESDAY	WEDNESDAY	THURSDAY
			1
5	6	7	8
12	13	14	15
19	20	21	22
26	27	28	29

May

2025

FRIDAY	SATURDAY	SUNDAY	NOTES
2	3	4	○
			○
			○
			○
			○
9	10	11	○
			○
			○
			○
16	17	18	○
			○
			○
			○
			○
23	24	25	○
			○
			○
			○
			○
30	31		NOTES

June

MONDAY	TUESDAY	WEDNESDAY	THURSDAY
2	3	4	5
9	10	11	12
16	17	18	19
23	24	25	26

June

FRIDAY	SATURDAY	SUNDAY	NOTES
		1	○
			○
			○
			○
			○
6	7	8	○
			○
			○
			○
13	14	15	○
			○
			○
			○
			○
20	21	22	○
			○
			○
			○
			○
27	28	29	30

July

2025

MONDAY	TUESDAY	WEDNESDAY	THURSDAY
	1	2	3
7	8	9	10
14	15	16	17
21	22	23	24
28	29	30	31

July

2025

FRIDAY	SATURDAY	SUNDAY	NOTES
4	5	6	○
			○
			○
			○
			○
11	12	13	○
			○
			○
			○
			○
18	19	20	○
			○
			○
			○
25	26	27	○
			○
			○
			○
			○
			NOTES

August 2025

MONDAY	TUESDAY	WEDNESDAY	THURSDAY
4	5	6	7
11	12	13	14
18	19	20	21
25	26	27	28

August 2025

FRIDAY	SATURDAY	SUNDAY	NOTES
1	2	3	○
			○
			○
			○
			○
8	9	10	○
			○
			○
			○
			○
15	16	17	○
			○
			○
			○
22	23	24	NOTES
29	30	31	

September 2025

MONDAY	TUESDAY	WEDNESDAY	THURSDAY
1	2	3	4
8	9	10	11
15	16	17	18
22	23	24	25
29	30		

September 2025

FRIDAY	SATURDAY	SUNDAY	NOTES
5	6	7	○
			○
			○
			○
			○
12	13	14	○
			○
			○
			○
			○
19	20	21	○
			○
			○
			○
26	27	28	○
			○
			○
			○
			○
			NOTES

October

MONDAY	TUESDAY	WEDNESDAY	THURSDAY
		1	2
6	7	8	9
13	14	15	16
20	21	22	23
27	28	29	30

October 2025

FRIDAY	SATURDAY	SUNDAY	NOTES
3	4	5	○
			○
			○
			○
			○
10	11	12	○
			○
			○
			○
			○
17	18	19	○
			○
			○
			○
24	25	26	○
			○
			○
			○
			○
31			NOTES

November 2025

MONDAY	TUESDAY	WEDNESDAY	THURSDAY
3	4	5	6
10	11	12	13
17	18	19	20
24	25	26	27

November 2025

FRIDAY	SATURDAY	SUNDAY	NOTES
	1	2	○
			○
			○
			○
			○
7	8	9	○
			○
			○
			○
			○
14	15	16	○
			○
			○
			○
21	22	23	○
			○
			○
			○
			○
28	29	30	NOTES

December 2025

THURSDAY	TUESDAY	WEDNESDAY	THURSDAY
1	2	3	4
8	9	10	11
15	16	17	18
22	23	24	25
29	30	31	

December

2025

FRIDAY	SATURDAY	SUNDAY	NOTES
5	6	7	○
			○
			○
			○
			○
12	13	14	○
			○
			○
			○
19	20	21	○
			○
			○
			○
			○
26	27	28	○
			○
			○
			○
			○
			NOTES

December
2024

01 SUNDAY

02 MONDAY

03 TUESDAY

04 WEDNESDAY

December
2024

05 THURSDAY

○
○
○
○
○
○
○
○

06 FRIDAY

○
○
○
○
○
○
○
○
○

07 SATURDAY

○
○
○
○
○
○
○
○

08 SUNDAY

○
○
○
○
○

09 MONDAY

○
○
○
○
○
○
○
○

10 TUESDAY

○
○
○
○
○
○
○
○

11 WEDNESDAY

○
○
○
○
○
○
○
○

12 THURSDAY

○
○
○
○
○

13 FRIDAY

○
○
○
○
○
○
○
○

14 SATURDAY

○
○
○
○
○
○
○
○
○

15 SUNDAY

○
○
○
○
○
○
○
○
○

16 MONDAY

○
○
○
○
○

17 TUESDAY

18 WEDNESDAY

19 THURSDAY

20 FRIDAY

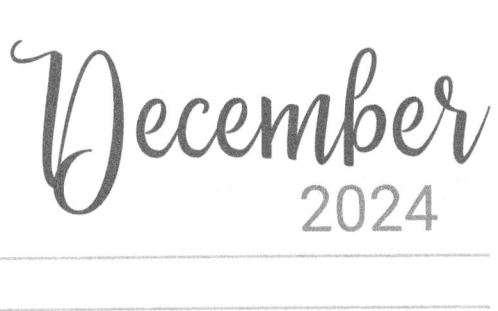

21 SATURDAY

○ _____
○ _____
○ _____
○ _____
○ _____
○ _____
○ _____
○ _____

22 SUNDAY

○ _____
○ _____
○ _____
○ _____
○ _____
○ _____
○ _____
○ _____

23 MONDAY

○ _____
○ _____
○ _____
○ _____
○ _____
○ _____
○ _____
○ _____

24 TUESDAY

○ _____
○ _____
○ _____
○ _____
○ _____

25 WEDNESDAY

○
○
○
○
○
○
○
○

26 THURSDAY

○
○
○
○
○
○
○
○

27 FRIDAY

○
○
○
○
○
○
○
○

28 SATURDAY

○
○
○
○
○

December
2024

29 SUNDAY

- ○
- ○
- ○
- ○
- ○
- ○
- ○
- ○

30 MONDAY

- ○
- ○
- ○
- ○
- ○
- ○
- ○
- ○

31 TUESDAY

- ○
- ○
- ○
- ○
- ○
- ○
- ○
- ○

NOTES

January 2025

01 WEDNESDAY

○
○
○
○
○
○
○
○

02 THURSDAY

○
○
○
○
○
○
○
○

03 FRIDAY

○
○
○
○
○
○
○
○

04 SATURDAY

○
○
○
○
○

January
2025

05 SUNDAY

○ _____
○ _____
○ _____
○ _____
○ _____
○ _____
○ _____
○ _____

06 MONDAY

○ _____
○ _____
○ _____
○ _____
○ _____
○ _____
○ _____
○ _____

07 TUESDAY

○ _____
○ _____
○ _____
○ _____
○ _____
○ _____
○ _____
○ _____

08 WEDNESDAY

○ _____
○ _____
○ _____
○ _____
○ _____

09 THURSDAY

10 FRIDAY

11 SATURDAY

12 SUNDAY

13 MONDAY

○
○
○
○
○
○
○
○

14 TUESDAY

○
○
○
○
○
○
○
○

15 WEDNESDAY

○
○
○
○
○
○
○
○

16 THURSDAY

○
○
○
○
○

17 FRIDAY

○
○
○
○
○
○
○
○

18 SATURDAY

○
○
○
○
○
○
○
○

19 SUNDAY

○
○
○
○
○
○
○
○

20 MONDAY

○
○
○
○
○

21 TUESDAY
○
○
○
○
○
○
○
○

22 WEDNESDAY
○
○
○
○
○
○
○
○

23 THURSDAY
○
○
○
○
○
○
○
○

24 FRIDAY
○
○
○
○
○

25 SATURDAY

○
○
○
○
○
○
○
○

26 SUNDAY

○
○
○
○
○
○
○
○

27 MONDAY

○
○
○
○
○
○
○
○

28 TUESDAY

○
○
○
○
○

29 WEDNESDAY

○ _____
○ _____
○ _____
○ _____
○ _____
○ _____
○ _____
○ _____

30 THURSDAY

○ _____
○ _____
○ _____
○ _____
○ _____
○ _____
○ _____
○ _____

31 FRIDAY

○ _____
○ _____
○ _____
○ _____
○ _____
○ _____
○ _____
○ _____

NOTES

_____
_____
_____
_____

February
2025

01 SATURDAY

02 SUNDAY

03 MONDAY

04 TUESDAY

February
2025

05 WEDNESDAY

○ _____
○ _____
○ _____
○ _____
○ _____
○ _____
○ _____
○ _____

06 THURSDAY

○ _____
○ _____
○ _____
○ _____
○ _____
○ _____
○ _____
○ _____

07 FRIDAY

○ _____
○ _____
○ _____
○ _____
○ _____
○ _____
○ _____
○ _____

08 SATURDAY

○ _____
○ _____
○ _____
○ _____
○ _____

February
2025

09 SUNDAY

○
○
○
○
○
○
○

10 MONDAY

○
○
○
○
○
○
○
○

11 TUESDAY

○
○
○
○
○
○
○
○

12 WEDNESDAY

○
○
○
○
○

February
2025

13 THURSDAY

○
○
○
○
○
○
○
○

14 FRIDAY

○
○
○
○
○
○
○
○

15 SATURDAY

○
○
○
○
○
○
○
○

16 SUNDAY

○
○
○
○
○

February
2025

17 MONDAY
○
○
○
○
○
○
○
○

18 TUESDAY
○
○
○
○
○
○
○
○

19 WEDNESDAY
○
○
○
○
○
○
○
○

20 THURSDAY
○
○
○
○
○

February 2025

21 FRIDAY

○ _____
○ _____
○ _____
○ _____
○ _____
○ _____
○ _____
○ _____

22 SATURDAY

○ _____
○ _____
○ _____
○ _____
○ _____
○ _____
○ _____
○ _____

23 SUNDAY

○ _____
○ _____
○ _____
○ _____
○ _____
○ _____
○ _____
○ _____

24 MONDAY

○ _____
○ _____
○ _____
○ _____
○ _____

25 TUESDAY

26 WEDNESDAY

27 THURSDAY

28 FRIDAY

March 2025

01 SATURDAY

○
○
○
○
○
○
○
○

02 SUNDAY

○
○
○
○
○
○
○
○

03 MONDAY

○
○
○
○
○
○
○
○

04 TUESDAY

○
○
○
○
○

March 2025

05 WEDNESDAY

06 THURSDAY

07 FRIDAY

08 SATURDAY

March
2025

09 SUNDAY

10 MONDAY

11 TUESDAY

12 WEDNESDAY

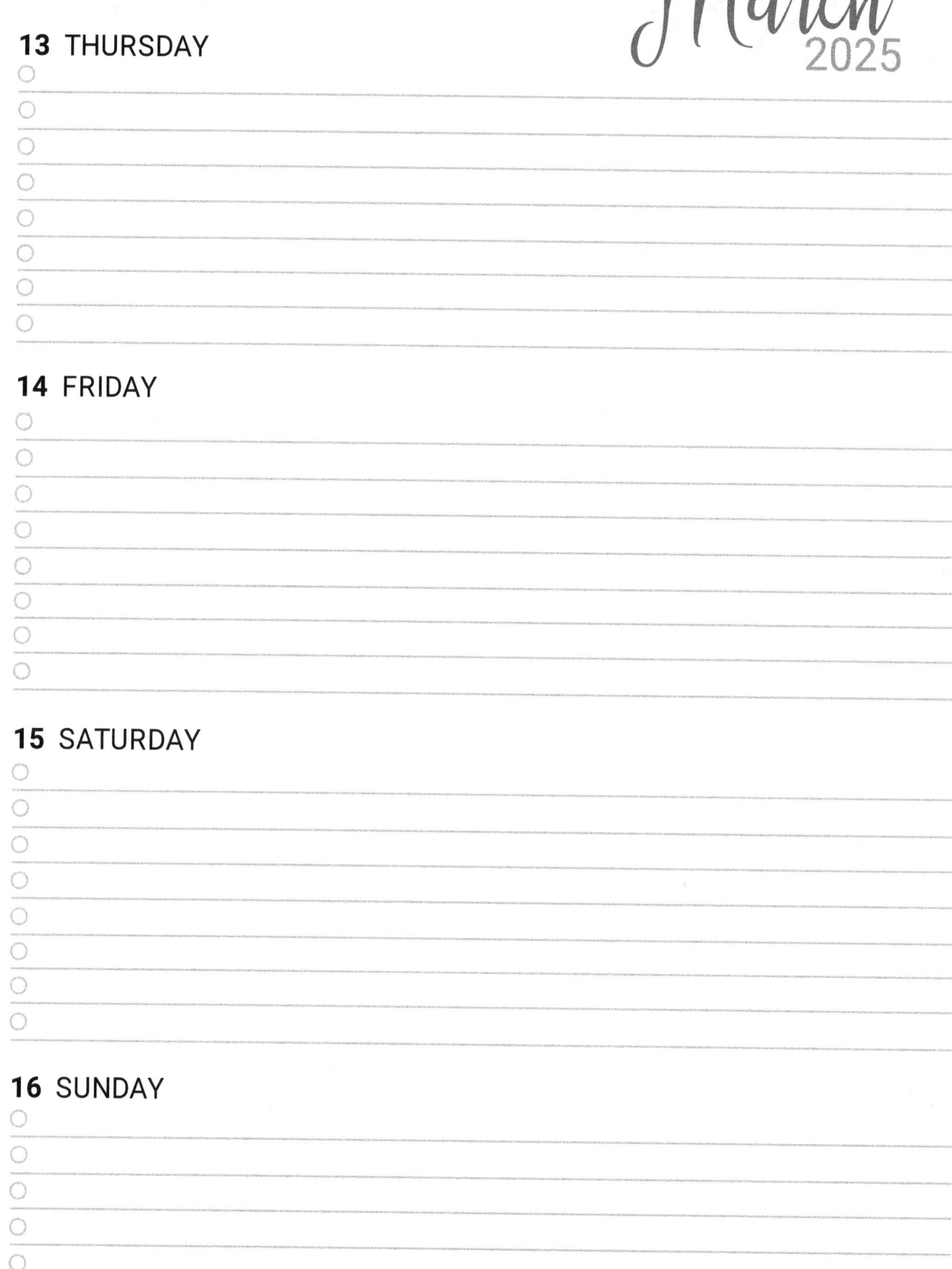

March
2025

13 THURSDAY

14 FRIDAY

15 SATURDAY

16 SUNDAY

March
2025

17 MONDAY
○
○
○
○
○
○
○
○

18 TUESDAY
○
○
○
○
○
○
○
○
○

19 WEDNESDAY
○
○
○
○
○
○
○
○

20 THURSDAY
○
○
○
○
○

21 FRIDAY

○
○
○
○
○
○
○
○

22 SATURDAY

○
○
○
○
○
○
○
○

23 SUNDAY

○
○
○
○
○
○
○
○

24 MONDAY

○
○
○
○
○

March
2025

25 TUESDAY

○ _____
○ _____
○ _____
○ _____
○ _____
○ _____
○ _____
○ _____

26 WEDNESDAY

○ _____
○ _____
○ _____
○ _____
○ _____
○ _____
○ _____
○ _____

27 THURSDAY

○ _____
○ _____
○ _____
○ _____
○ _____
○ _____
○ _____
○ _____

28 FRIDAY

○ _____
○ _____
○ _____
○ _____
○ _____

March
2025

29 SATURDAY

○ _____
○ _____
○ _____
○ _____
○ _____
○ _____
○ _____
○ _____

30 SUNDAY

○ _____
○ _____
○ _____
○ _____
○ _____
○ _____
○ _____
○ _____

31 MONDAY

○ _____
○ _____
○ _____
○ _____
○ _____
○ _____
○ _____
○ _____

NOTES

_____
_____
_____
_____

April
2025

01 TUESDAY

○
○
○
○
○
○
○

02 WEDNESDAY

○
○
○
○
○
○
○
○

03 THURSDAY

○
○
○
○
○
○
○
○

04 FRIDAY

○
○
○
○
○

05 SATURDAY

06 SUNDAY

07 MONDAY

08 TUESDAY

April
2025

09 WEDNESDAY

○
○
○
○
○
○
○
○

10 THURSDAY

○
○
○
○
○
○
○
○

11 FRIDAY

○
○
○
○
○
○
○
○

12 SATURDAY

○
○
○
○
○

April
2025

13 SUNDAY

14 MONDAY

15 TUESDAY

16 WEDNESDAY

April
2025

17 THURSDAY

○

○

○

○

○

○

○

18 FRIDAY

○

○

○

○

○

○

○

○

19 SATURDAY

○

○

○

○

○

○

○

○

20 SUNDAY

○

○

○

○

○

21 MONDAY

22 TUESDAY

23 WEDNESDAY

24 THURSDAY

April
2025

25 FRIDAY
○
○
○
○
○
○
○

26 SATURDAY
○
○
○
○
○
○
○
○

27 SUNDAY
○
○
○
○
○
○
○
○

28 MONDAY
○
○
○
○
○

April
2025

29 TUESDAY

○
○
○
○
○
○
○
○

30 WEDNESDAY

○
○
○
○
○
○
○
○

NOTES

May
2025

01 THURSDAY
○
○
○
○
○
○
○

02 FRIDAY
○
○
○
○
○
○
○

03 SATURDAY
○
○
○
○
○
○
○

04 SUNDAY
○
○
○
○
○

May
2025

05 MONDAY

06 TUESDAY

07 WEDNESDAY

08 THURSDAY

09 FRIDAY

○ ─────────────────────────────
○ ─────────────────────────────
○ ─────────────────────────────
○ ─────────────────────────────
○ ─────────────────────────────
○ ─────────────────────────────
○ ─────────────────────────────
○ ─────────────────────────────

10 SATURDAY

○ ─────────────────────────────
○ ─────────────────────────────
○ ─────────────────────────────
○ ─────────────────────────────
○ ─────────────────────────────
○ ─────────────────────────────
○ ─────────────────────────────
○ ─────────────────────────────

11 SUNDAY

○ ─────────────────────────────
○ ─────────────────────────────
○ ─────────────────────────────
○ ─────────────────────────────
○ ─────────────────────────────
○ ─────────────────────────────
○ ─────────────────────────────
○ ─────────────────────────────

12 MONDAY

○ ─────────────────────────────
○ ─────────────────────────────
○ ─────────────────────────────
○ ─────────────────────────────
○ ─────────────────────────────

May
2025

13 TUESDAY

○
○
○
○
○
○
○
○

14 WEDNESDAY

○
○
○
○
○
○
○
○

15 THURSDAY

○
○
○
○
○
○
○
○

16 FRIDAY

○
○
○
○
○

17 SATURDAY

○
○
○
○
○
○
○
○

18 SUNDAY

○
○
○
○
○
○
○
○
○

19 MONDAY

○
○
○
○
○
○
○
○

20 TUESDAY

○
○
○
○
○

May
2025

21 WEDNESDAY

22 THURSDAY

23 FRIDAY

24 SATURDAY

25 SUNDAY

○ _____
○ _____
○ _____
○ _____
○ _____
○ _____
○ _____
○ _____

26 MONDAY

○ _____
○ _____
○ _____
○ _____
○ _____
○ _____
○ _____
○ _____

27 TUESDAY

○ _____
○ _____
○ _____
○ _____
○ _____
○ _____
○ _____
○ _____

28 WEDNESDAY

○ _____
○ _____
○ _____
○ _____
○ _____

May
2025

29 THURSDAY
○
○
○
○
○
○
○
○

30 FRIDAY
○
○
○
○
○
○
○
○

31 SATURDAY
○
○
○
○
○
○
○
○

NOTES

June 2025

01 SUNDAY

○ _____
○ _____
○ _____
○ _____
○ _____
○ _____
○ _____
○ _____

02 MONDAY

○ _____
○ _____
○ _____
○ _____
○ _____
○ _____
○ _____
○ _____

03 TUESDAY

○ _____
○ _____
○ _____
○ _____
○ _____
○ _____
○ _____
○ _____

04 WEDNESDAY

○ _____
○ _____
○ _____
○ _____
○ _____

June
2025

05 THURSDAY

06 FRIDAY

07 SATURDAY

08 SUNDAY

June
2025

09 MONDAY
- ◯
- ◯
- ◯
- ◯
- ◯
- ◯
- ◯
- ◯

10 TUESDAY
- ◯
- ◯
- ◯
- ◯
- ◯
- ◯
- ◯
- ◯

11 WEDNESDAY
- ◯
- ◯
- ◯
- ◯
- ◯
- ◯
- ◯
- ◯

12 THURSDAY
- ◯
- ◯
- ◯
- ◯
- ◯

13 FRIDAY

○
○
○
○
○
○
○
○

14 SATURDAY

○
○
○
○
○
○
○
○

15 SUNDAY

○
○
○
○
○
○
○
○

16 MONDAY

○
○
○
○
○

17 TUESDAY

○
○
○
○
○
○
○
○

18 WEDNESDAY

○
○
○
○
○
○
○
○

19 THURSDAY

○
○
○
○
○
○
○
○

20 FRIDAY

○
○
○
○
○

21 SATURDAY

22 SUNDAY

23 MONDAY

24 TUESDAY

25 WEDNESDAY

○ _____
○ _____
○ _____
○ _____
○ _____
○ _____
○ _____
○ _____

26 THURSDAY

○ _____
○ _____
○ _____
○ _____
○ _____
○ _____
○ _____
○ _____

27 FRIDAY

○ _____
○ _____
○ _____
○ _____
○ _____
○ _____
○ _____
○ _____

28 SATURDAY

○ _____
○ _____
○ _____
○ _____
○ _____

29 SUNDAY

○ _____
○ _____
○ _____
○ _____
○ _____
○ _____
○ _____
○ _____

30 MONDAY

○ _____
○ _____
○ _____
○ _____
○ _____
○ _____
○ _____
○ _____

NOTES

_____
_____
_____
_____
_____
_____
_____
_____
_____
_____
_____
_____

July

2025

01 TUESDAY

○
○
○
○
○
○
○
○

02 WEDNESDAY

○
○
○
○
○
○
○
○
○

03 THURSDAY

○
○
○
○
○
○
○
○
○

04 FRIDAY

○
○
○
○
○

July
2025

05 SATURDAY

06 SUNDAY

07 MONDAY

08 TUESDAY

09 WEDNESDAY

10 THURSDAY

11 FRIDAY

12 SATURDAY

July
2025

13 SUNDAY

14 MONDAY

15 TUESDAY

16 WEDNESDAY

July
2025

17 THURSDAY

18 FRIDAY

19 SATURDAY

20 SUNDAY

July

21 MONDAY

22 TUESDAY

23 WEDNESDAY

24 THURSDAY

July
2025

25 FRIDAY
- ○
- ○
- ○
- ○
- ○
- ○
- ○
- ○

26 SATURDAY
- ○
- ○
- ○
- ○
- ○
- ○
- ○
- ○
- ○

27 SUNDAY
- ○
- ○
- ○
- ○
- ○
- ○
- ○
- ○

28 MONDAY
- ○
- ○
- ○
- ○
- ○

29 TUESDAY

○ _____
○ _____
○ _____
○ _____
○ _____
○ _____
○ _____
○ _____

30 WEDNESDAY

○ _____
○ _____
○ _____
○ _____
○ _____
○ _____
○ _____
○ _____

31 THURSDAY

○ _____
○ _____
○ _____
○ _____
○ _____
○ _____
○ _____
○ _____

NOTES

_____
_____
_____
_____

August
2025

01 FRIDAY

- ○
- ○
- ○
- ○
- ○
- ○
- ○
- ○

02 SATURDAY

- ○
- ○
- ○
- ○
- ○
- ○
- ○
- ○

03 SUNDAY

- ○
- ○
- ○
- ○
- ○
- ○
- ○
- ○

04 MONDAY

- ○
- ○
- ○
- ○
- ○

05 TUESDAY

○
○
○
○
○
○
○
○

06 WEDNESDAY

○
○
○
○
○
○
○
○

07 THURSDAY

○
○
○
○
○
○
○
○

08 FRIDAY

○
○
○
○
○

09 SATURDAY

○
○
○
○
○
○
○
○

10 SUNDAY

○
○
○
○
○
○
○
○

11 MONDAY

○
○
○
○
○
○
○
○

12 TUESDAY

○
○
○
○
○

August
2025

13 WEDNESDAY

14 THURSDAY

15 FRIDAY

16 SATURDAY

17 SUNDAY

○
○
○
○
○
○
○
○

18 MONDAY

○
○
○
○
○
○
○
○

19 TUESDAY

○
○
○
○
○
○
○
○

20 WEDNESDAY

○
○
○
○
○

21 THURSDAY

22 FRIDAY

23 SATURDAY

24 SUNDAY

25 MONDAY
○
○
○
○
○
○
○
○

26 TUESDAY
○
○
○
○
○
○
○
○
○

27 WEDNESDAY
○
○
○
○
○
○
○
○

28 THURSDAY
○
○
○
○
○

29 FRIDAY

○
○
○
○
○
○
○
○

30 SATURDAY

○
○
○
○
○
○
○
○

31 SUNDAY

○
○
○
○
○
○
○
○

NOTES

September
2025

01 MONDAY

○ _____
○ _____
○ _____
○ _____
○ _____
○ _____
○ _____
○ _____

02 TUESDAY

○ _____
○ _____
○ _____
○ _____
○ _____
○ _____
○ _____
○ _____

03 WEDNESDAY

○ _____
○ _____
○ _____
○ _____
○ _____
○ _____
○ _____
○ _____

04 THURSDAY

○ _____
○ _____
○ _____
○ _____
○ _____

September
2025

05 FRIDAY

○
○
○
○
○
○
○
○

06 SATURDAY

○
○
○
○
○
○
○
○

07 SUNDAY

○
○
○
○
○
○
○
○

08 MONDAY

○
○
○
○
○

09 TUESDAY

○ ─────────────────────────────
○ ─────────────────────────────
○ ─────────────────────────────
○ ─────────────────────────────
○ ─────────────────────────────
○ ─────────────────────────────
○ ─────────────────────────────
○ ─────────────────────────────

10 WEDNESDAY

○ ─────────────────────────────
○ ─────────────────────────────
○ ─────────────────────────────
○ ─────────────────────────────
○ ─────────────────────────────
○ ─────────────────────────────
○ ─────────────────────────────
○ ─────────────────────────────

11 THURSDAY

○ ─────────────────────────────
○ ─────────────────────────────
○ ─────────────────────────────
○ ─────────────────────────────
○ ─────────────────────────────
○ ─────────────────────────────
○ ─────────────────────────────
○ ─────────────────────────────

12 FRIDAY

○ ─────────────────────────────
○ ─────────────────────────────
○ ─────────────────────────────
○ ─────────────────────────────
○ ─────────────────────────────

13 SATURDAY

○
○
○
○
○
○
○
○

14 SUNDAY

○
○
○
○
○
○
○
○

15 MONDAY

○
○
○
○
○
○
○
○

16 TUESDAY

○
○
○
○
○

17 WEDNESDAY

○ _____
○ _____
○ _____
○ _____
○ _____
○ _____
○ _____

18 THURSDAY

○ _____
○ _____
○ _____
○ _____
○ _____
○ _____
○ _____
○ _____

19 FRIDAY

○ _____
○ _____
○ _____
○ _____
○ _____
○ _____
○ _____
○ _____

20 SATURDAY

○ _____
○ _____
○ _____
○ _____
○ _____

21 SUNDAY

○
○
○
○
○
○
○
○

22 MONDAY

○
○
○
○
○
○
○
○

23 TUESDAY

○
○
○
○
○
○
○
○

24 WEDNESDAY

○
○
○
○
○

25 THURSDAY

○ _____
○ _____
○ _____
○ _____
○ _____
○ _____
○ _____
○ _____

26 FRIDAY

○ _____
○ _____
○ _____
○ _____
○ _____
○ _____
○ _____
○ _____

27 SATURDAY

○ _____
○ _____
○ _____
○ _____
○ _____
○ _____
○ _____
○ _____

28 SUNDAY

○ _____
○ _____
○ _____
○ _____
○ _____

29 MONDAY

○ _____
○ _____
○ _____
○ _____
○ _____
○ _____
○ _____
○ _____

30 TUESDAY

○ _____
○ _____
○ _____
○ _____
○ _____
○ _____
○ _____
○ _____

NOTES

_____
_____
_____
_____
_____
_____
_____
_____
_____
_____

01 WEDNESDAY

○
○
○
○
○
○
○
○

02 THURSDAY

○
○
○
○
○
○
○
○
○

03 FRIDAY

○
○
○
○
○
○
○
○

04 SATURDAY

○
○
○
○
○

October
2025

05 SUNDAY

06 MONDAY

07 TUESDAY

08 WEDNESDAY

09 THURSDAY

○
○
○
○
○
○
○
○

10 FRIDAY

○
○
○
○
○
○
○
○

11 SATURDAY

○
○
○
○
○
○
○
○

12 SUNDAY

○
○
○
○
○

13 MONDAY

14 TUESDAY

15 WEDNESDAY

16 THURSDAY

October
2025

17 FRIDAY
○
○
○
○
○
○
○
○

18 SATURDAY
○
○
○
○
○
○
○
○

19 SUNDAY
○
○
○
○
○
○
○
○

20 MONDAY
○
○
○
○
○

October
2025

21 TUESDAY

○
○
○
○
○
○
○
○

22 WEDNESDAY

○
○
○
○
○
○
○
○

23 THURSDAY

○
○
○
○
○
○
○
○

24 FRIDAY

○
○
○
○
○

25 SATURDAY

○ _____
○ _____
○ _____
○ _____
○ _____
○ _____
○ _____
○ _____

26 SUNDAY

○ _____
○ _____
○ _____
○ _____
○ _____
○ _____
○ _____
○ _____

27 MONDAY

○ _____
○ _____
○ _____
○ _____
○ _____
○ _____
○ _____
○ _____

28 TUESDAY

○ _____
○ _____
○ _____
○ _____
○ _____

October
2025

29 WEDNESDAY

30 THURSDAY

31 FRIDAY

NOTES

November
2025

01 SATURDAY

○
○
○
○
○
○
○
○

02 SUNDAY

○
○
○
○
○
○
○
○

03 MONDAY

○
○
○
○
○
○
○
○

04 TUESDAY

○
○
○
○
○

05 WEDNESDAY

06 THURSDAY

07 FRIDAY

08 SATURDAY

09 SUNDAY

○
○
○
○
○
○
○
○

10 MONDAY

○
○
○
○
○
○
○
○

11 TUESDAY

○
○
○
○
○
○
○
○

12 WEDNESDAY

○
○
○
○
○

13 THURSDAY

○
○
○
○
○
○
○
○

14 FRIDAY

○
○
○
○
○
○
○
○

15 SATURDAY

○
○
○
○
○
○
○
○

16 SUNDAY

○
○
○
○
○

November
2025

17 MONDAY

18 TUESDAY

19 WEDNESDAY

20 THURSDAY

November
2025

21 FRIDAY
○
○
○
○
○
○
○
○

22 SATURDAY
○
○
○
○
○
○
○
○

23 SUNDAY
○
○
○
○
○
○
○
○

24 MONDAY
○
○
○
○
○

25 TUESDAY

○ _____
○ _____
○ _____
○ _____
○ _____
○ _____
○ _____
○ _____

26 WEDNESDAY

○ _____
○ _____
○ _____
○ _____
○ _____
○ _____
○ _____
○ _____

27 THURSDAY

○ _____
○ _____
○ _____
○ _____
○ _____
○ _____
○ _____
○ _____

28 FRIDAY

○ _____
○ _____
○ _____
○ _____
○ _____

29 SATURDAY
○ _____
○ _____
○ _____
○ _____
○ _____
○ _____
○ _____
○ _____

30 SUNDAY
○ _____
○ _____
○ _____
○ _____
○ _____
○ _____
○ _____
○ _____

NOTES

December
2025

01 MONDAY

○ _____
○ _____
○ _____
○ _____
○ _____
○ _____
○ _____
○ _____

02 TUESDAY

○ _____
○ _____
○ _____
○ _____
○ _____
○ _____
○ _____
○ _____

03 WEDNESDAY

○ _____
○ _____
○ _____
○ _____
○ _____
○ _____
○ _____
○ _____

04 THURSDAY

○ _____
○ _____
○ _____
○ _____
○ _____

05 FRIDAY

06 SATURDAY

07 SUNDAY

08 MONDAY

December
2025

09 TUESDAY
○
○
○
○
○
○
○
○

10 WEDNESDAY
○
○
○
○
○
○
○
○
○

11 THURSDAY
○
○
○
○
○
○
○
○
○

12 FRIDAY
○
○
○
○
○

13 SATURDAY

14 SUNDAY

15 MONDAY

16 TUESDAY

17 WEDNESDAY

○
○
○
○
○
○
○
○

18 THURSDAY

○
○
○
○
○
○
○
○

19 FRIDAY

○
○
○
○
○
○
○
○

20 SATURDAY

○
○
○
○
○

21 SUNDAY

○
○
○
○
○
○
○
○

22 MONDAY

○
○
○
○
○
○
○
○

23 TUESDAY

○
○
○
○
○
○
○
○

24 WEDNESDAY

○
○
○
○
○

25 THURSDAY
- ○
- ○
- ○
- ○
- ○
- ○
- ○
- ○

26 FRIDAY
- ○
- ○
- ○
- ○
- ○
- ○
- ○
- ○

27 SATURDAY
- ○
- ○
- ○
- ○
- ○
- ○
- ○
- ○

28 SUNDAY
- ○
- ○
- ○
- ○
- ○

December
2025

29 MONDAY

30 TUESDAY

31 WEDNESDAY

NOTES

www.ingramcontent.com/pod-product-compliance
Lightning Source LLC
Chambersburg PA
CBHW081332120626
46546CB00011B/3318